PEOPLE AT WORK

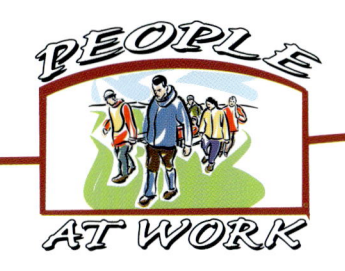

IN
MOUNTAIN RESCUE

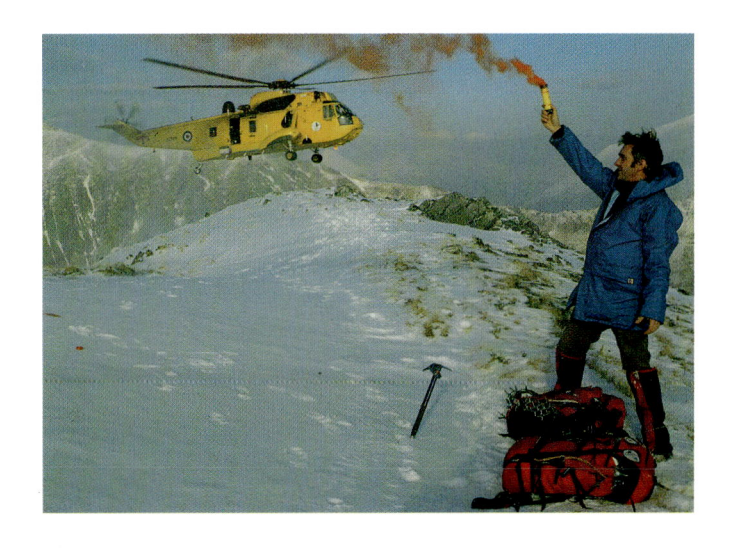

DEBORAH FOX

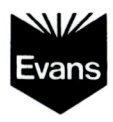

Evans

EVANS BROTHERS LIMITED

Published by Evans Brothers Limited
2a Portman Mansions
Chiltern Street
London
W1M 1LE

© 1998 Evans Brothers Limited

First published in 1998

All rights reserved. No part of this publication may be reproduced, stored in a retrieval system or transmitted in any form or by any means, electronic, mechanical, photocopying, recording or otherwise, without prior permission of Evans Brothers Limited.

Commissioned by: Su Swallow
Design: Neil Sayer
Photographer: Alan Towse
Illustrator: Liam Bonney/The Art Market

British Library Cataloguing in Publication Data

Fox, Deborah
 People at work in mountain rescue
 1.Mountaineering - Search and rescue operations - Juvenile literature
 I.Title
 363.1'4

ISBN 0237518260

Printed in Hong Kong by Wing King Tong

Acknowledgements

The author and publisher wish to thank the following for their help:
Justin Squires and the Edale Mountain Rescue team; Brian Williamson and the Kinder Mountain Rescue team;
Dr P.J. Andrew of the Mountain Rescue Council; Alex Gillespie and Miller Harris of the Lochaber Mountain Rescue team; Malcolm Bowyer, Alex Muller and Mike Amps of the Search and Rescue Dogs Association (SARDA), Norma Muller, and Holly, Glyn and Trigg.

We would like to thank the following for permission to reproduce the following photographs: Alex Gillespie Photography cover (top right), title page, pages 19 (bottom), 22, 23, 24, and 25.

Contents

The team	8
Preparation	10
Finding the casualty	12
Looking after the casualty	14
Winching up	16
Search and rescue dogs	18
Out on a search	20
Snow and ice	22
In an emergency	24
De-briefing	26
Glossary	28
Index	29

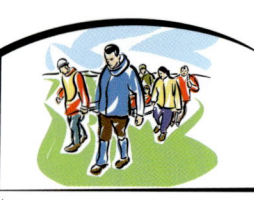

The team

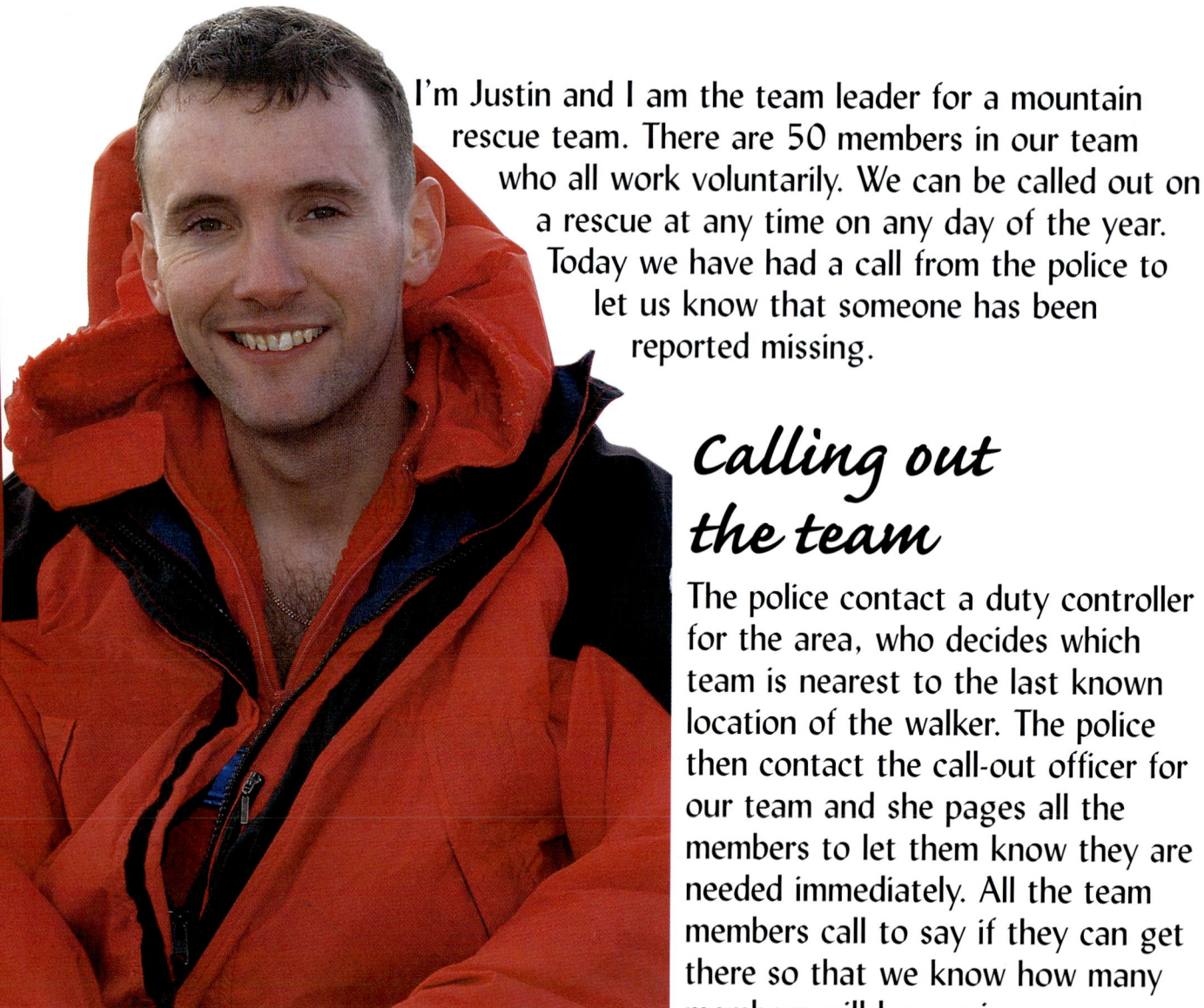

I'm Justin and I am the team leader for a mountain rescue team. There are 50 members in our team who all work voluntarily. We can be called out on a rescue at any time on any day of the year. Today we have had a call from the police to let us know that someone has been reported missing.

Calling out the team

The police contact a duty controller for the area, who decides which team is nearest to the last known location of the walker. The police then contact the call-out officer for our team and she pages all the members to let them know they are needed immediately. All the team members call to say if they can get there so that we know how many members will be coming.

Working from base

Some teams work from a base where they keep all their equipment and the radios. All the team members meet, or rendezvous, at the base. Each team has its own controller who coordinates and manages the rescue.

▲ The team looks at the area it is covering for the rescue.

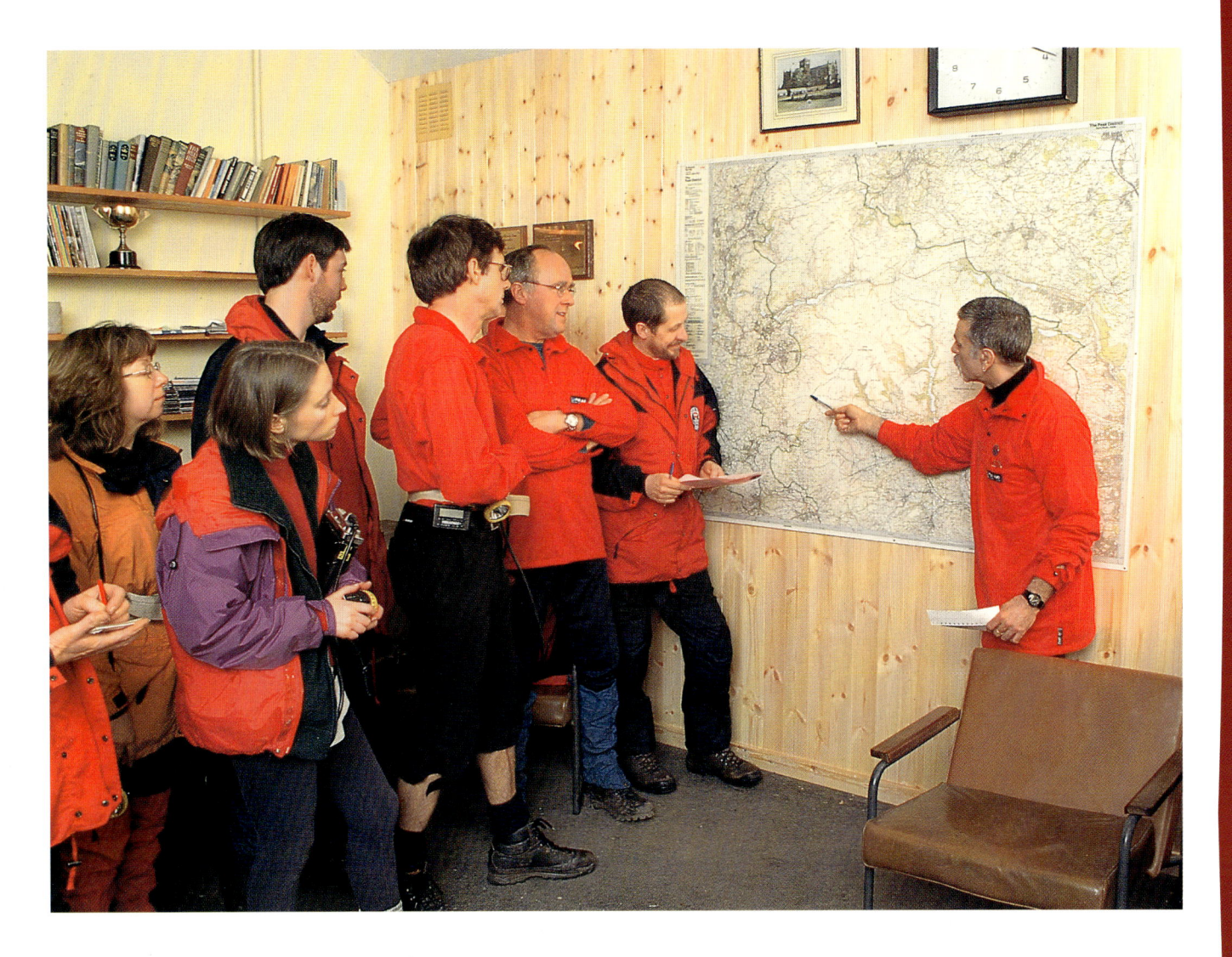

Working from a vehicle

Some rescue teams work from a four-wheel drive vehicle, keeping all the equipment in the back. When we already know where the casualty is, the call-out officer tells us to meet at the vehicle, which will be as close as possible to the casualty. This can save a lot of time.

I have been a member of the team for about eight years, training on the job. I have always been a keen walker and climber. As a team leader I need to know the area and the abilities of all the team members well.

9

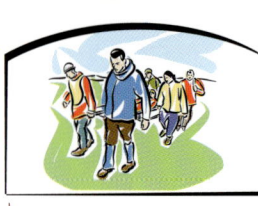

Preparation

The controller's job, like the team leader's, is based on experience. I think of all the facts I can gather together to make the team's job easier. We have a form with a list of questions on missing people, such as whether the person has asthma or any allergies. I try to piece together all the details ... is the walker well equipped, does he or she have any medical problems, and did that person take a car and, if so, where is it parked?

Ted, controller

One of the team does a radio check to make sure communications to the police, the ambulance service and the helicopter team are all working properly. I talk to the controller about how we should approach the rescue.

The controller

The controller stays at the base to coordinate and support the team. If a team is searching for a casualty, the

▼ *Communication is the most important aspect of any rescue.*

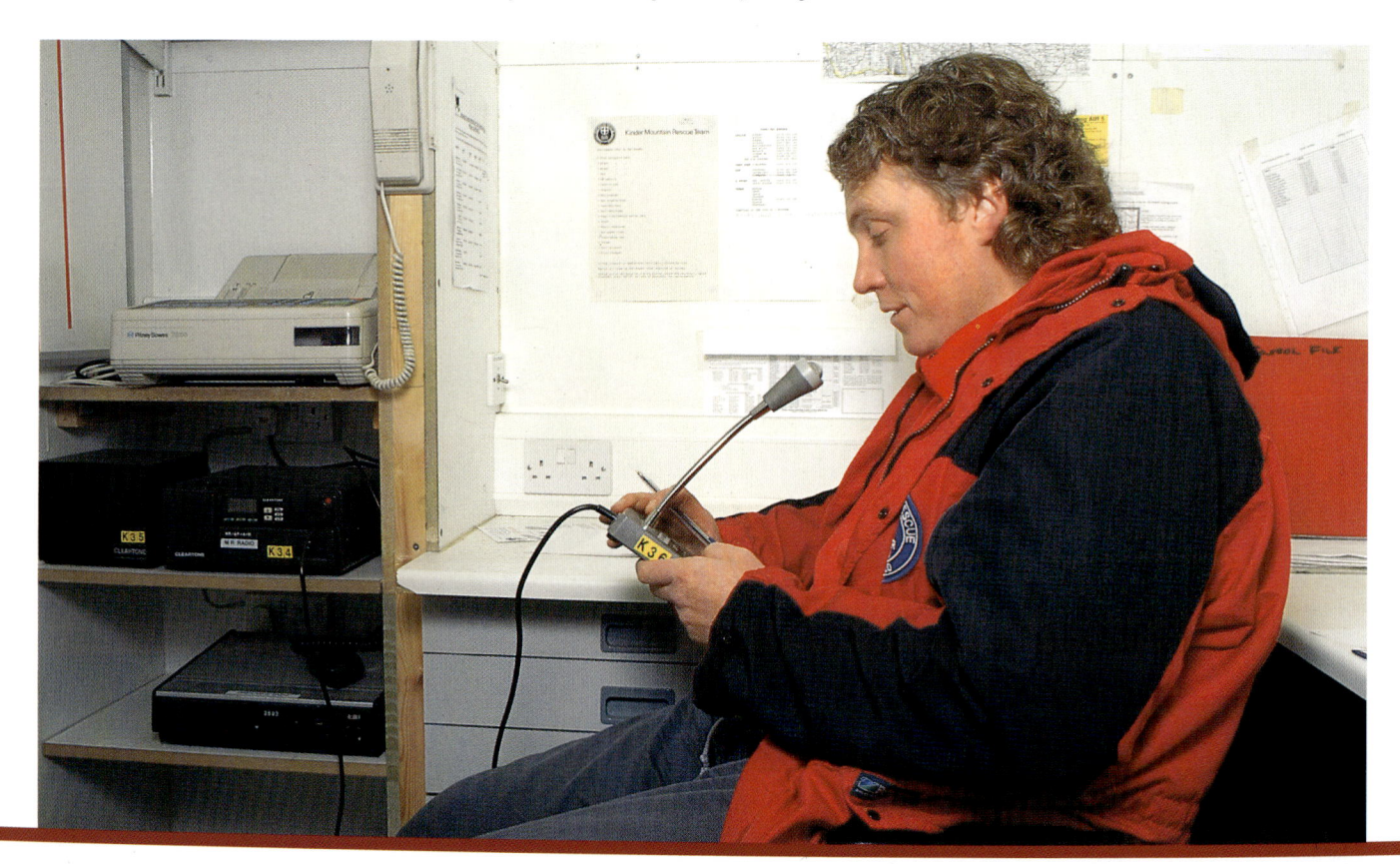

▶ This is some of the equipment we wear and carry. Clockwise: helmet, gloves, ropes and harness, crampons, gaiters, ice axe, sling (purple), notebook, compass, map, global positioning system and strobe light.

controller tries to find out as much as possible about that person and thinks of factors that will make the team's job easier. For example, if there is a strong wind in the area, the controller doesn't want to make us walk straight into the wind as this will slow us down.

Equipment

There is a huge amount of equipment needed by every team – for first aid and for climbing. We carry ropes and climbing gear, a tent, search lamps, flares, medical kits, pagers, binoculars, food and warm, waterproof clothing. Each member needs to be able to carry equipment weighing about 18 kilogrammes and so we all need to be fit.

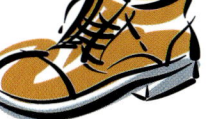

First aid equipment
- Stretcher to carry patients
- Backboard for spinal injury
- Neck collars
- Splints for broken bones
- Resuscitation masks and oxygen cylinders
- Thermometer for diagnosing hypothermia
- Casualty bag to keep patient warm
- Vacuum mattress to keep person rigid on the stretcher

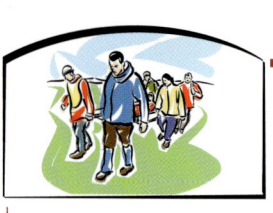

Finding the casualty

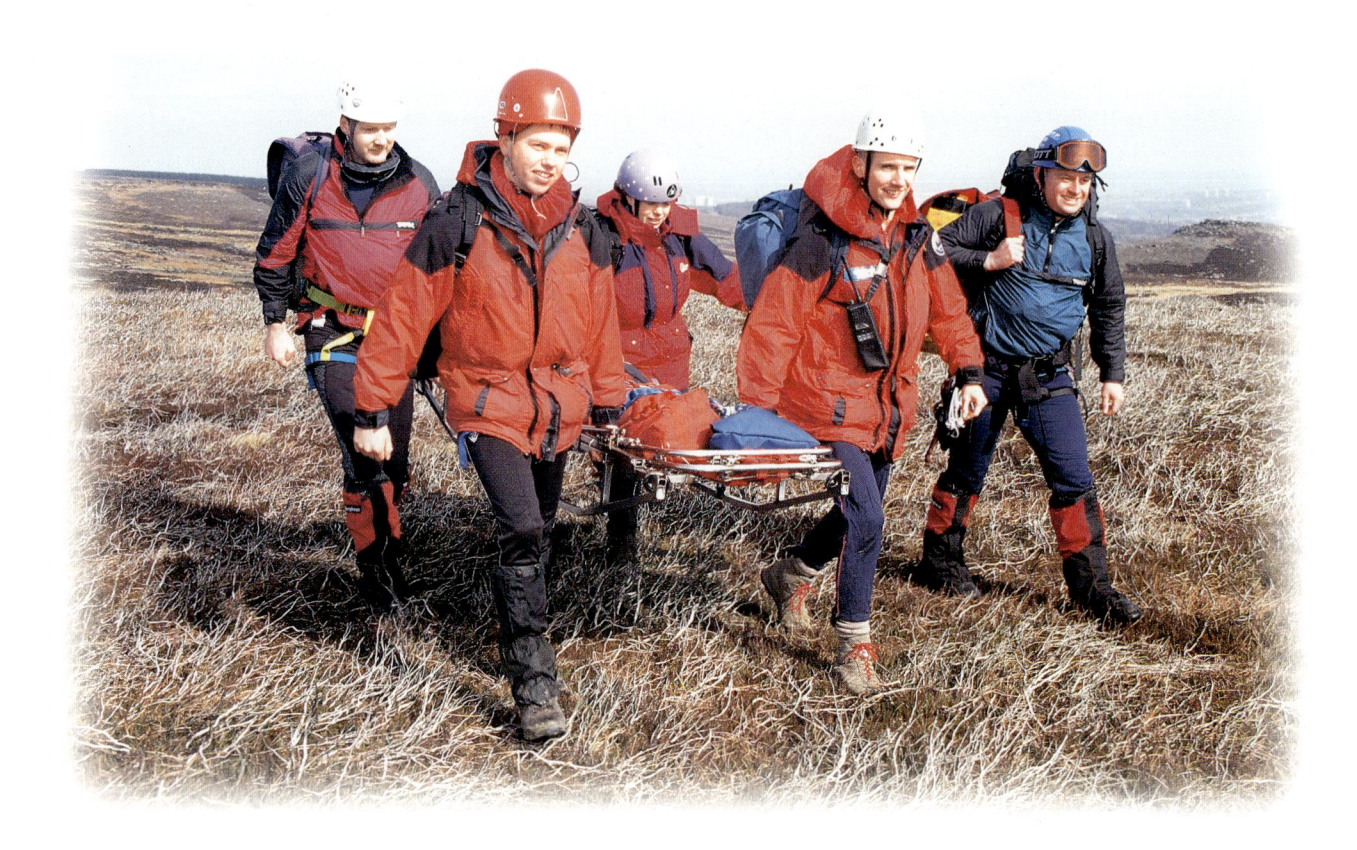

We train on weekends throughout the year and on certain evenings during the week in all kinds of weather conditions – snow, ice, wind and rain. We all know how to use the radios, how to navigate and map-read, how to use all the equipment and how to give first aid.

Neil, training officer

I brief everyone on the area we are covering and where we think the casualty might be. Checking our maps and carrying equipment, we set off to the last known location of the walker. As the weather is fairly clear this makes our rescue much easier. If we have to search at night or in bad weather then it is so much more difficult. After two

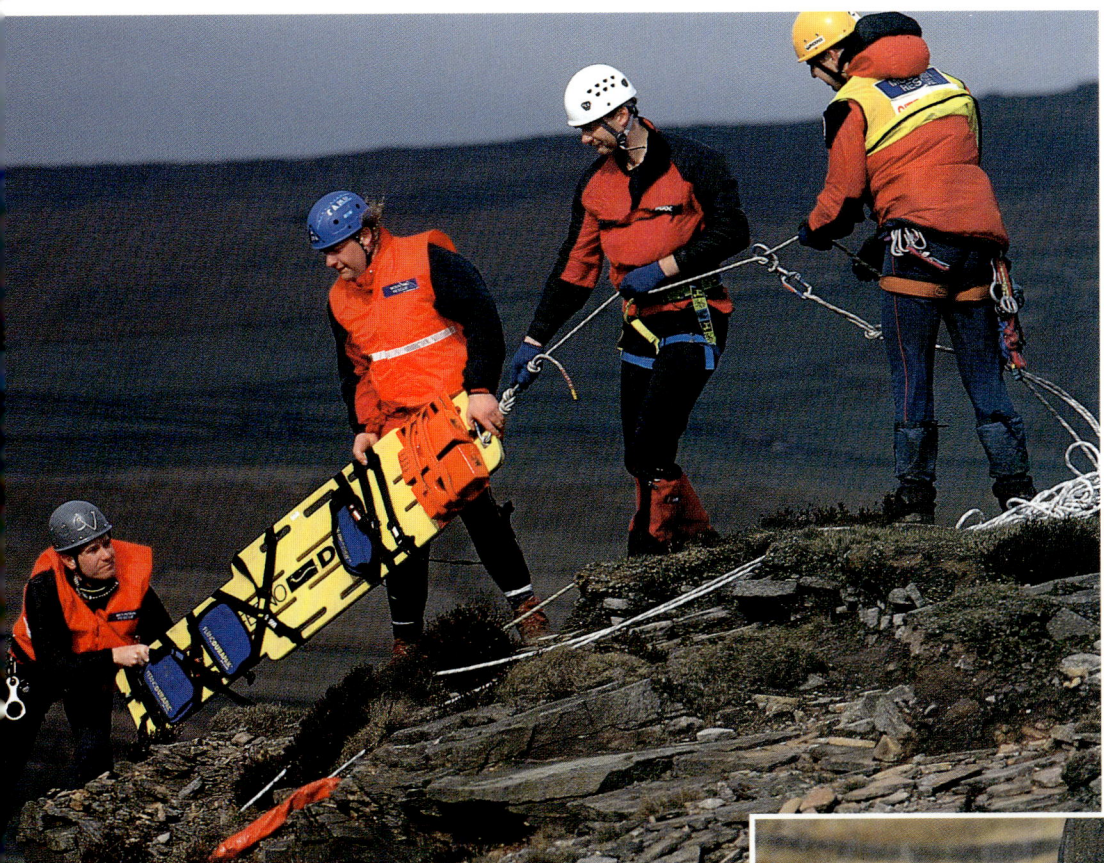

◀ *Several members of the team pass equipment to the members who are on the ledge with the casualty.*

hours I radio back to the controller to let him know that we have found the casualty and will assess if he has any injuries.

Securing ropes

The casualty is lying on a ledge. We need to get down to him quickly. We tie the ropes to metal stakes to make sure that they are quite firm. All the team members are trained in how to use ropes and in the use of knots.

▶ *One member lowers himself to the ledge.*

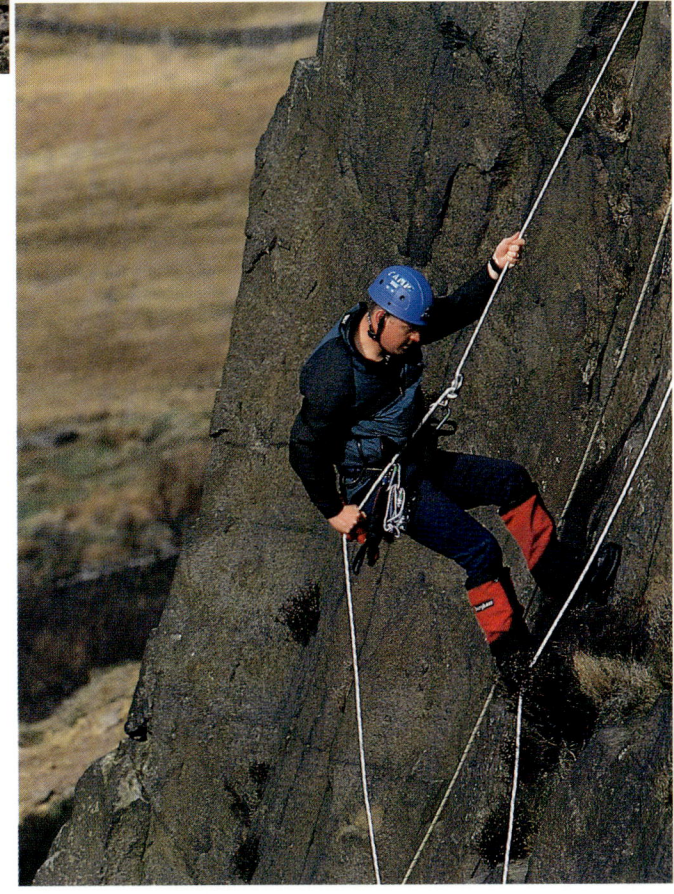

13

Looking after the casualty

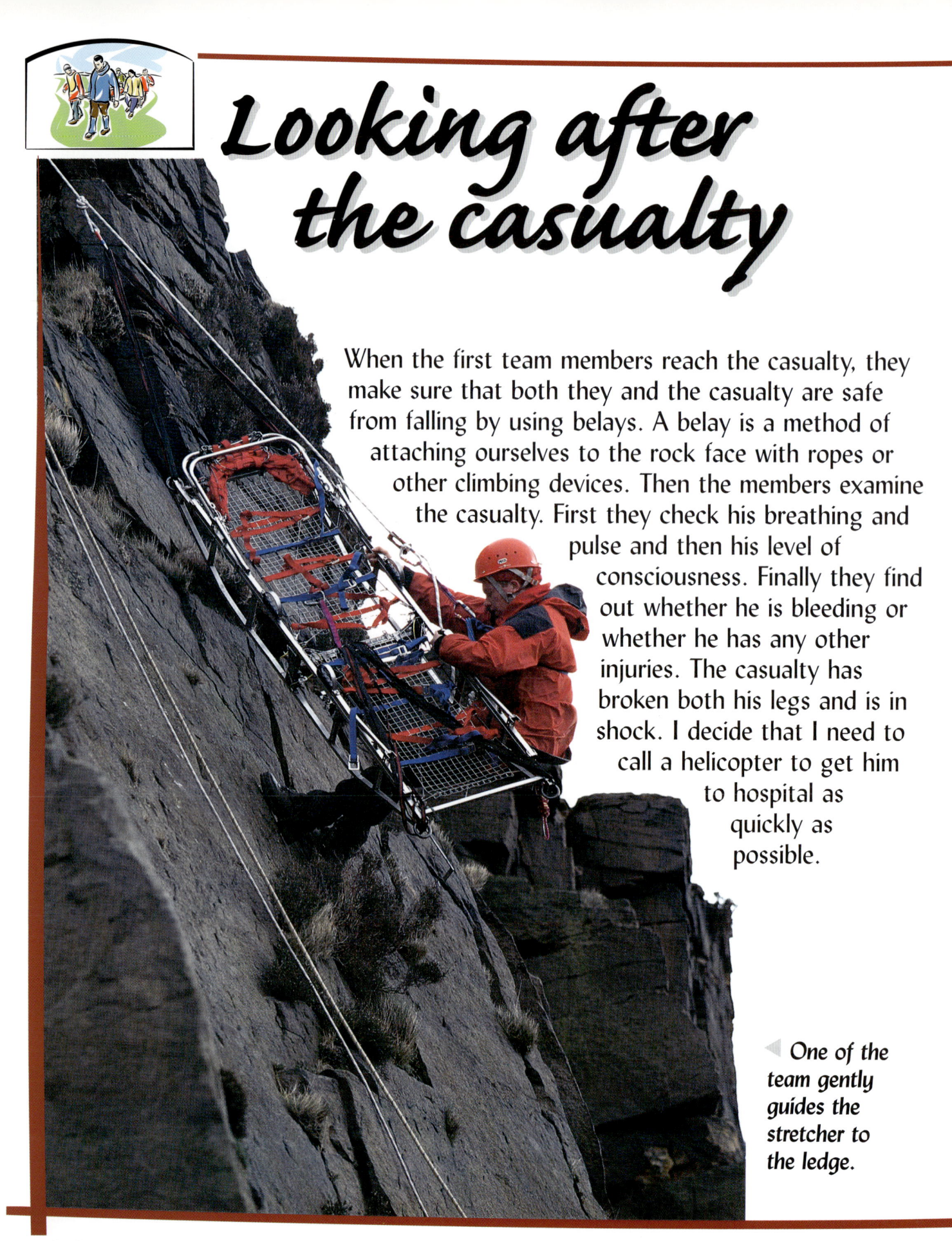

When the first team members reach the casualty, they make sure that both they and the casualty are safe from falling by using belays. A belay is a method of attaching ourselves to the rock face with ropes or other climbing devices. Then the members examine the casualty. First they check his breathing and pulse and then his level of consciousness. Finally they find out whether he is bleeding or whether he has any other injuries. The casualty has broken both his legs and is in shock. I decide that I need to call a helicopter to get him to hospital as quickly as possible.

◀ *One of the team gently guides the stretcher to the ledge.*

▶ If there is a doctor in the team, the doctor can give the patient intravenous fluid to replace any blood that has been lost or to treat shock.

Using the stretcher

One of the team guides the stretcher as we lower it to the ledge. We set the legs in box splints and keep the patient warm by wrapping him in a casualty bag. It is important to keep the patient warm to avoid any risk of hypothermia. We keep checking on his condition to make sure he is stable.

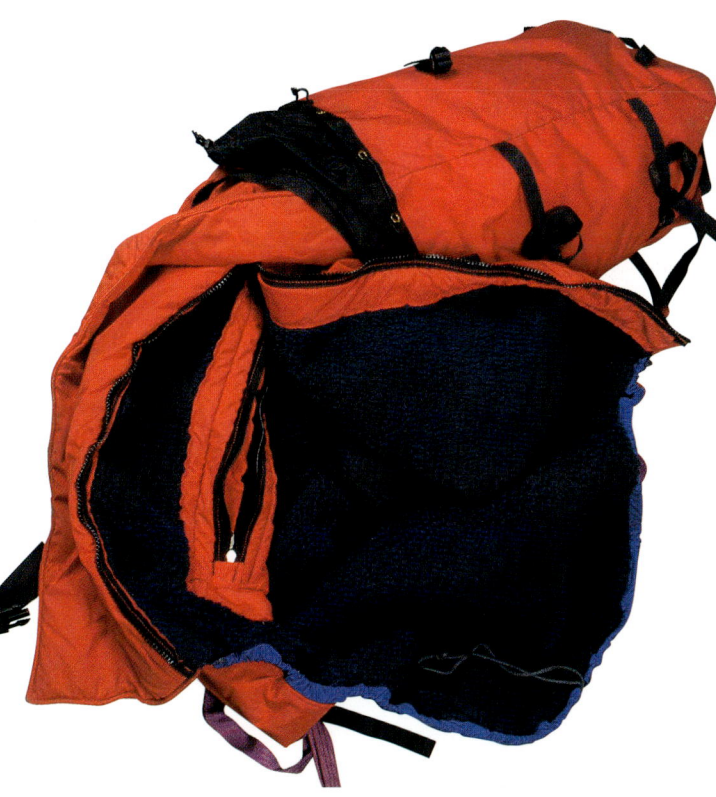

▲ The casualty bag is a waterproof, fleece-lined sleeping bag that gives extra insulation against the wind.

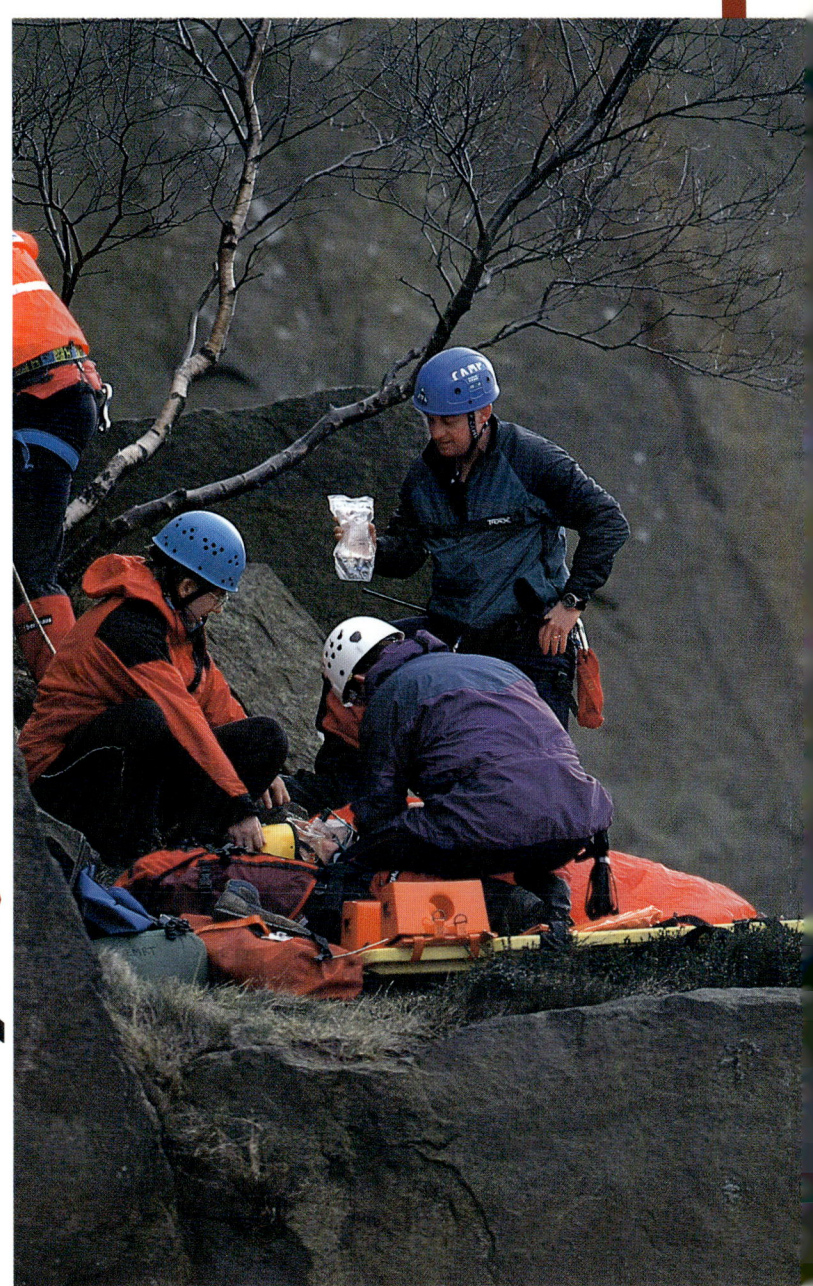

Although we happen to have two doctors in our team, we are all qualified in first aid and are examined on it every three years. We can all apply splints to broken legs, check blood pressure and we know how to treat hypothermia.

Stephanie, team member

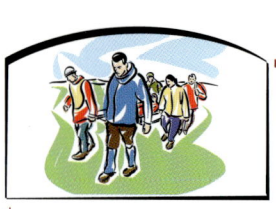

Winching up

The helicopter crew arrives and the pilot circles the area to assess how strong the winds are. He has to decide whether he can land or whether to winch up the casualty to the helicopter. The winchman sits in a special harness, which is secured to a steel cable, and he is gently lowered to the casualty. He attaches the stretcher to the cable and gives a signal for the winch operator to start winching up.

> We are all trained paramedics. When you save people who are in hostile environments and in danger of losing their lives, it's an amazing feeling.
>
> Trevor, winchman

▼ The helicopter pilot keeps a careful eye on the instruments as he stays in the hover position.

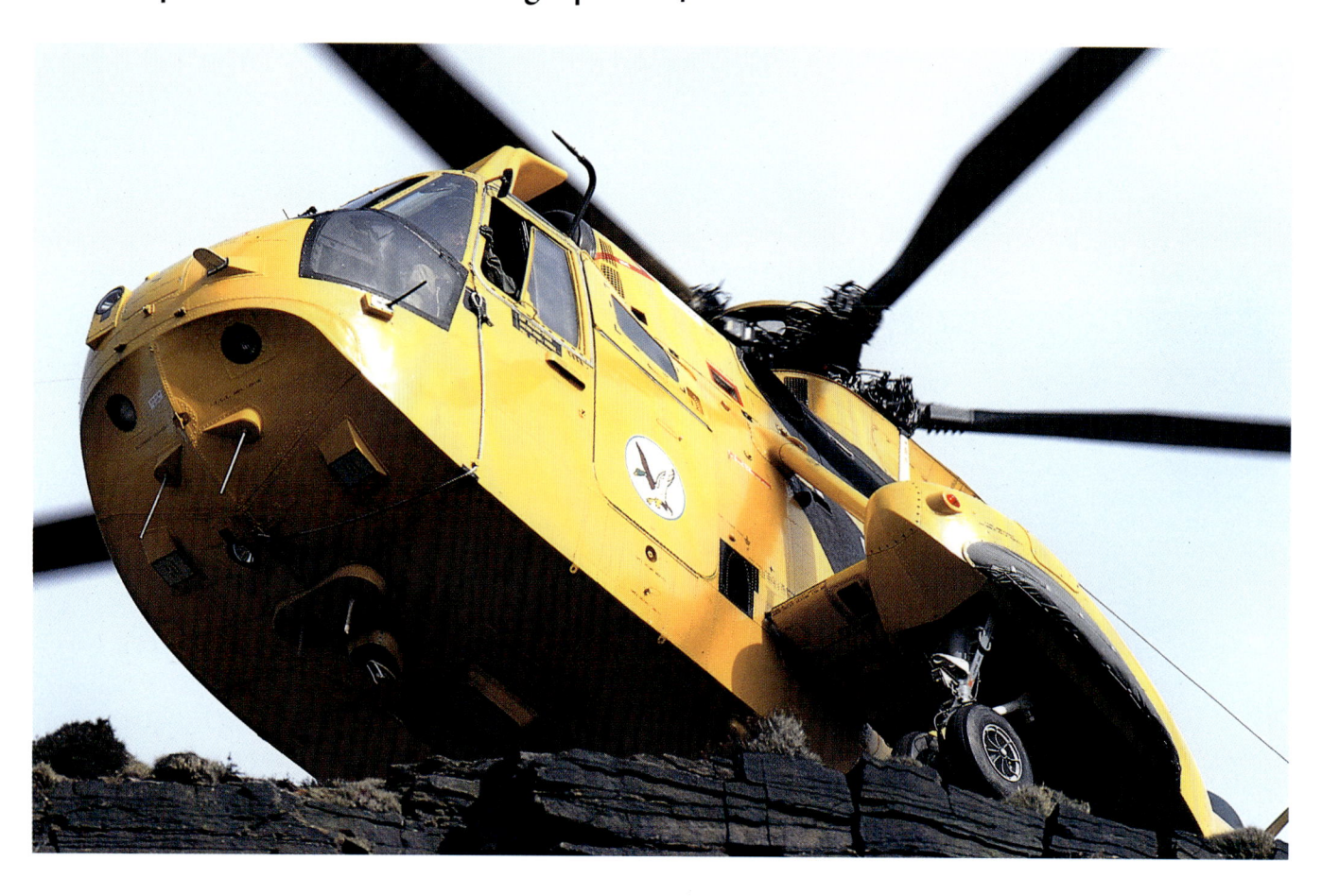

▶ Here the winchman sits in a special harness. He uses hand signals to tell the winch operator when he should stop winching and when to restart so that the stretcher is moved smoothly and steadily.

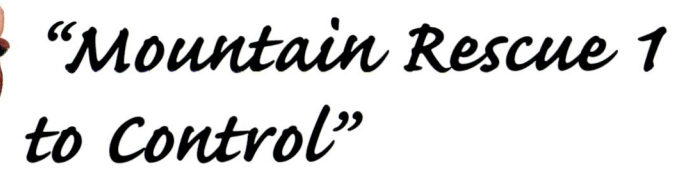

"Mountain Rescue 1 to Control"

As the helicopter takes the patient to hospital, I make a radio call to the controller to let him know what has happened. He makes sure the ambulance is waiting for the helicopter. We pack up the ropes and all the equipment we have used. If anything is wet, we need to dry it out before the next rescue.

We have to make sure we are properly dressed to keep ourselves warm as well as the casualty. Temperatures can drop to -20°C with the wind chill.

Nick, team member

Search and rescue dogs

For some rescues it is useful to call out search and rescue dogs and their handlers, particularly at night and in bad weather. The dogs are trained to use air scent to find missing people.

Training

The dogs start training when they are puppies, at about eight or nine weeks old. It takes about two and a half years to train the dogs before they are allowed to go out on searches.

> I looked for an inquisitive puppy, one that looked alert, with bright eyes and his ears pricking up. Trigg is a good strong puppy.
>
> Malcolm, instructor

> It can take up to nine months to get a dog fully trained in obedience. It's a big commitment for people to take on and they have to be sure they can devote the time to the training. Training has got to be a joy to a new handler.
>
> Malcolm, instructor

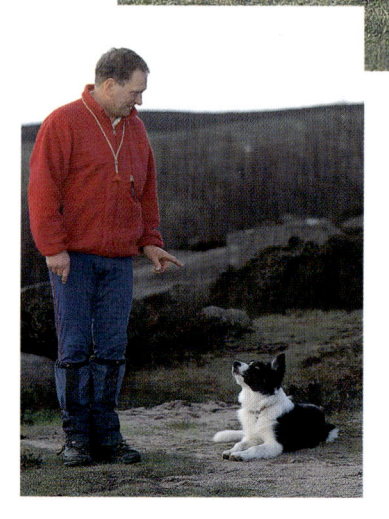

▲ Trigg learns how to walk close to Malcolm's heel.

◄ Trigg is taught the 'downstay'.

The handler starts the training by playing little games with the puppy. Then the puppy has to learn how to be obedient – how to sit and stay and how to walk at the handler's heel. The dog has to learn to do a 'downstay', which means that he must stay on the ground for ten minutes. If the dog moves, he fails the obedience test.

Ice and snow

Rescue dogs can also use their sense of smell to detect people who are buried under snow. A dog's sense of smell is said to be hundreds of times greater than a human's. When the dog detects human scent he lets his owner know, usually by barking. When he makes a find, the dog paws at the snow.

Praising the dog

It is important to acknowledge and encourage search dogs. They love to work and to them searching is a game. The dog handlers give lots of praise to their dogs when they find the casualties and reward them with their favourite toys or biscuits.

▼ *This search dog finds the casualty who is buried in the snow, but still conscious.*

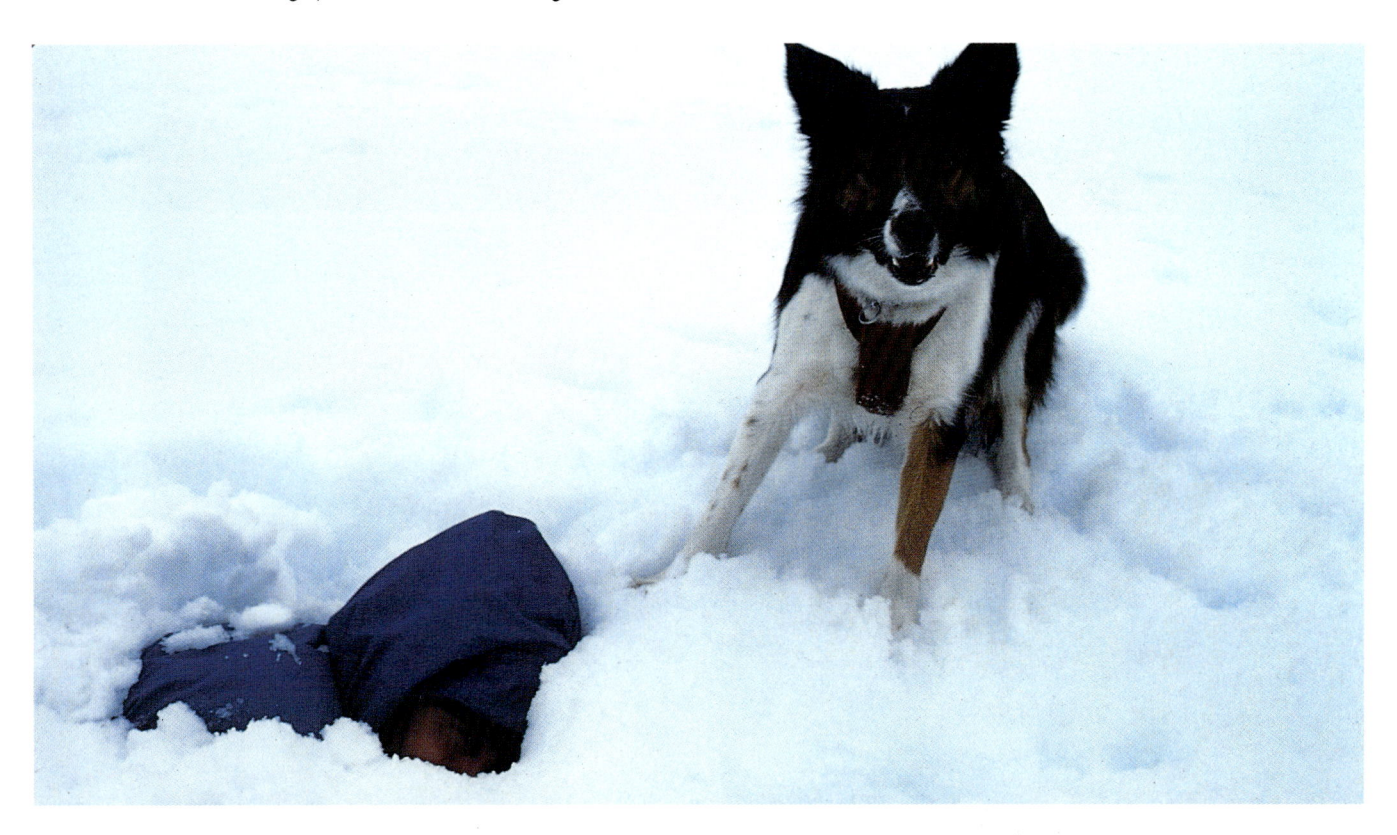

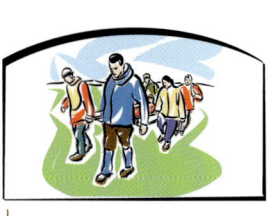

Out on a search

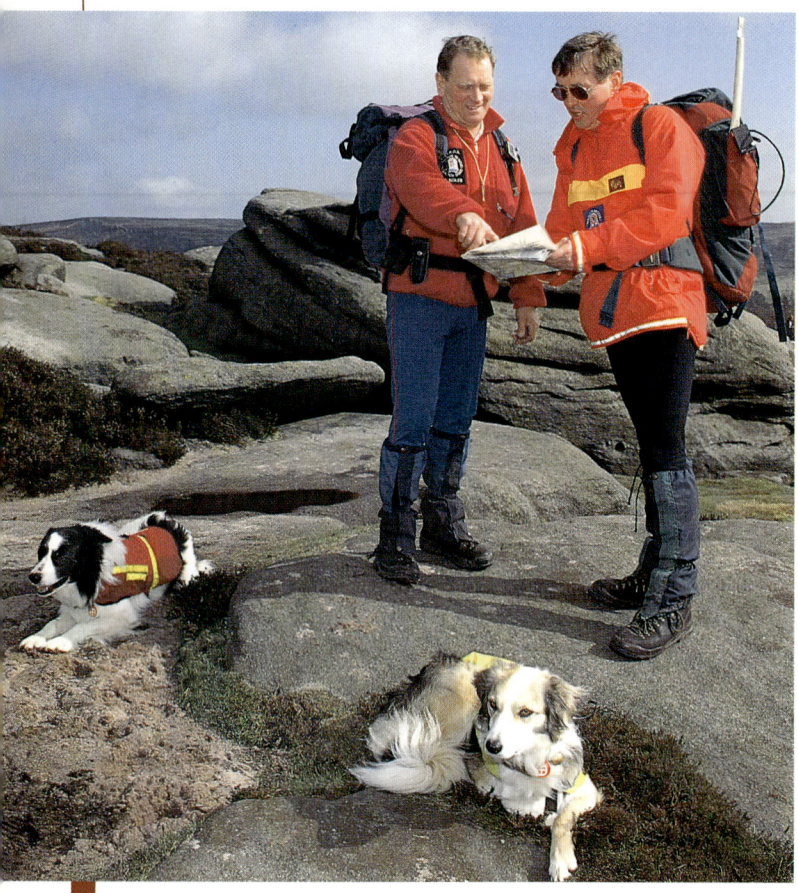

▲ Before the search, the handlers check their position on the map.

▼ The handler, Alex, prepares Holly for the search.

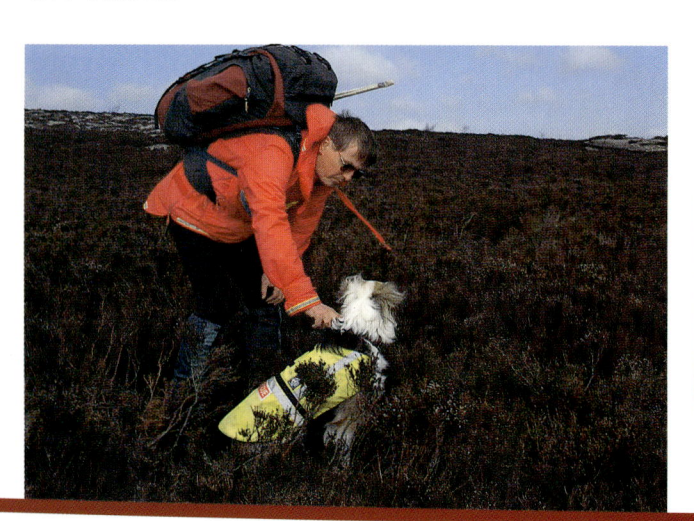

The team controller gives the dog handlers areas to search and it is up to the handler to make sure the area is covered. The handler works with the dog making sure the instructions to the dog are clear, such as "Find" and "Show me". The handler works the dog across the wind, which makes it easier for the dog to pick up human scent. When the dog picks up a scent he will run off in that direction, coming back to lead the handler the same way. As the dog continues the search, the handler always encourages the dog, saying "Show me, show me".

Finding the casualty

After two hours Holly has picked up the scent and leads her handler, Alex, to the missing person. Alex praises Holly. He then radios the rest of the team to let them know the condition of the casualty and their location. He

> When Holly finds the casualty, she puts her nose up close to make sure she has followed the scent to its source.
>
> Alex, handler

20

makes sure the casualty is kept warm until the team arrive to carry the stretcher to a waiting ambulance. Sometimes a dog can pick up the wrong human scent and if this happens, the handler simply instructs the dog to start searching again. Usually though, the missing person is in a remote location.

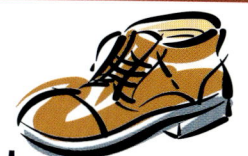

Dog signals

Handlers use a combination of signals to instruct their dogs – voice commands, whistles, and hand and arm signals. The signals are to tell the dog to find, to move left and right, and a recall signal.

▶ Holly stands next to the casualty leading Alex to her.

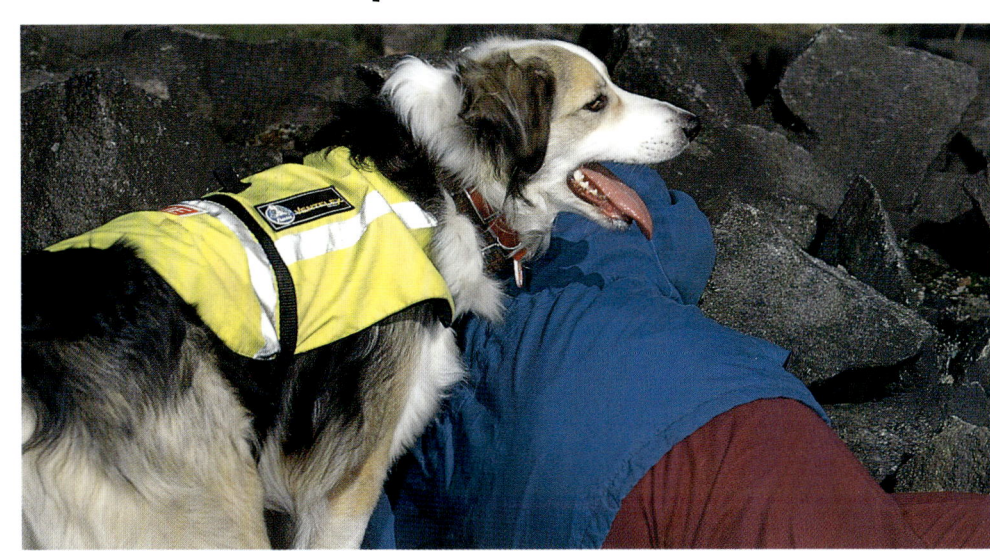

▼ Our team carries the casualty to the ambulance.

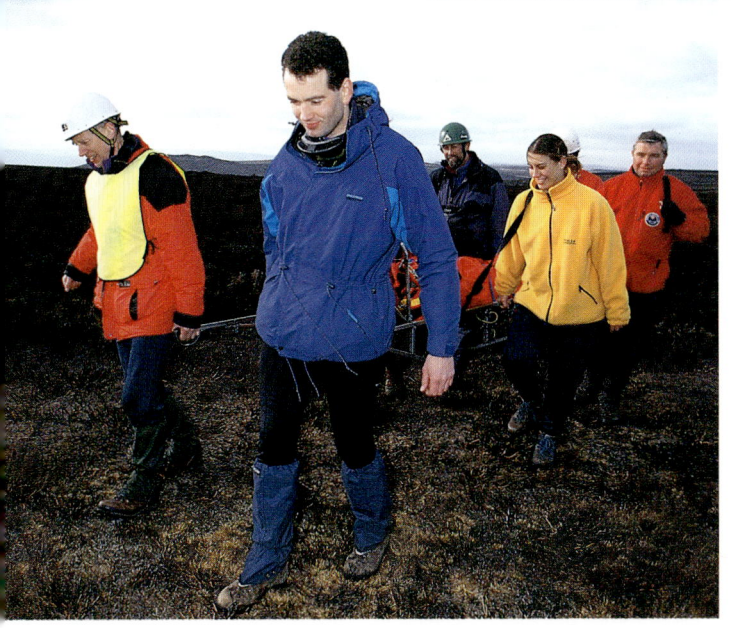

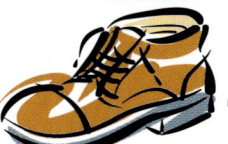

Air and ground scent

Some police dogs use ground scent to find missing people, but the disadvantage is that this method can lengthen the search. The dogs follow a ground scent and if the person has walked round in circles, the dogs will follow the same trail as the person. With air scent the dog moves directly towards the person.

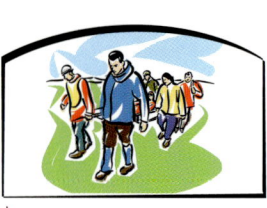

Snow and ice

In bad weather or in snow and ice, mountain rescue teams have to be well equipped to deal with the extreme conditions. All the members of the team carry ice axes and attach crampons to their boots, which provide extra grip in the ice and snow.

A team has been called out to locate a missing person who has been reported missing from a mountain climb. Visibility isn't good as the snow has fallen thickly. The team set off, but need to keep close together.

After four hours the weather clears a little and the team spot the casualty in a gully. It is important to keep him warm and so they wrap him in a bivouac bag. They need to assess his medical condition. He is breathing

> If a strong wind blows then it is hard to see in the 'spindrift'. Usually we get a blast of this and then the snow settles as the wind drops.
>
> Alex, team member

▼ It is important that team members keep sight of one another when visibility is bad.

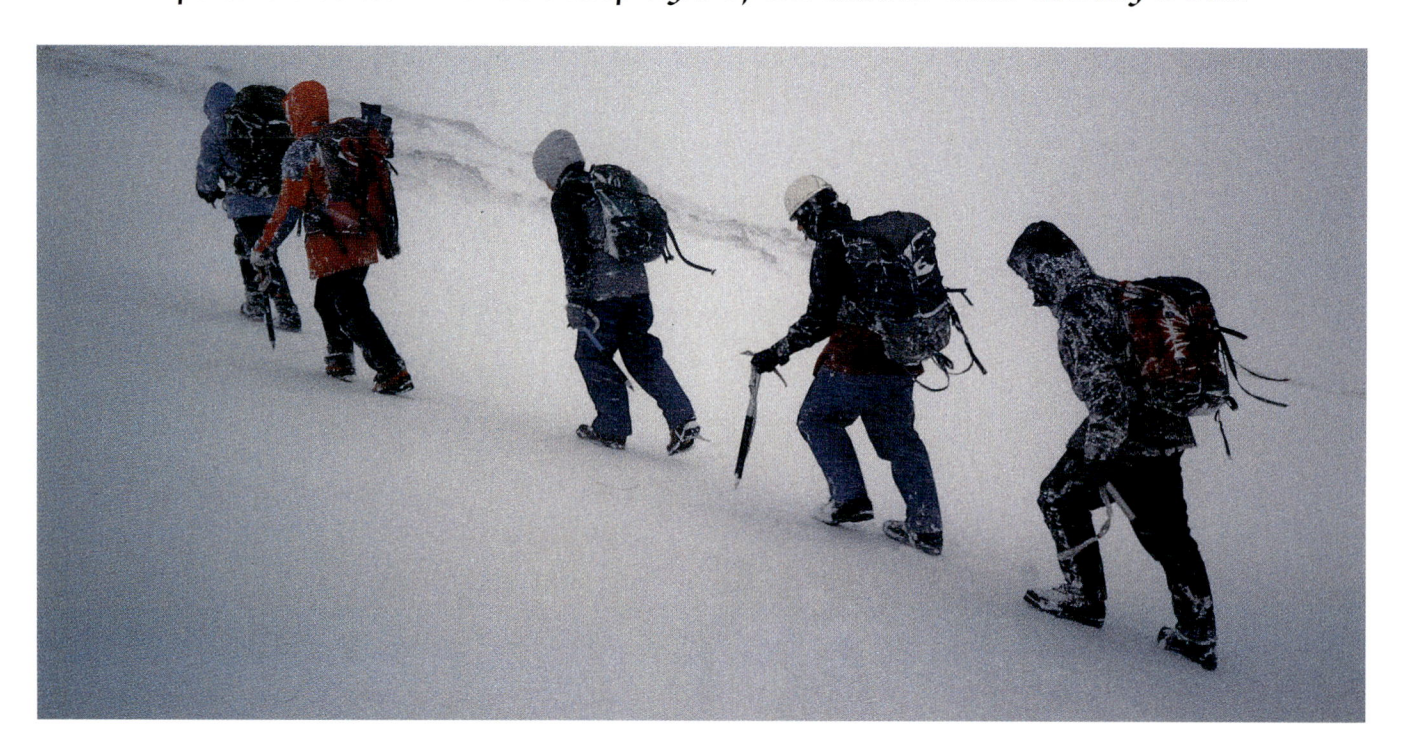

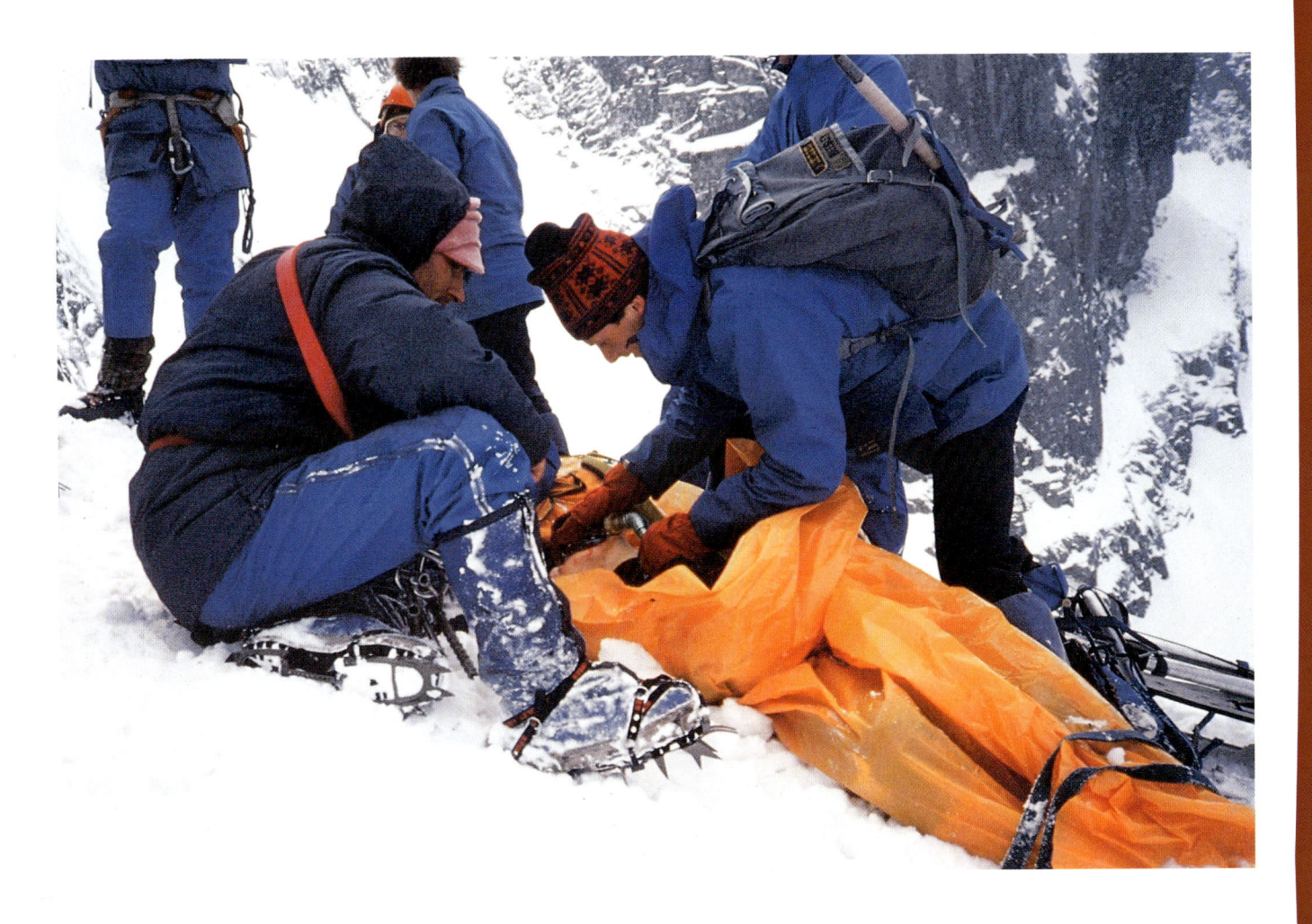

After hitting his head and breaking his ankle, the climber is suffering from exhaustion, mild hypothermia and shock.

rapidly and is pale and cold, which could indicate shock. Severely shocked patients are often given oxygen.

Lowering the stretcher

Two members of the team tie the stretcher to themselves to keep it secure because it could easily slide down the mountain. They need to keep the casualty as steady as possible as they take him to an ambulance.

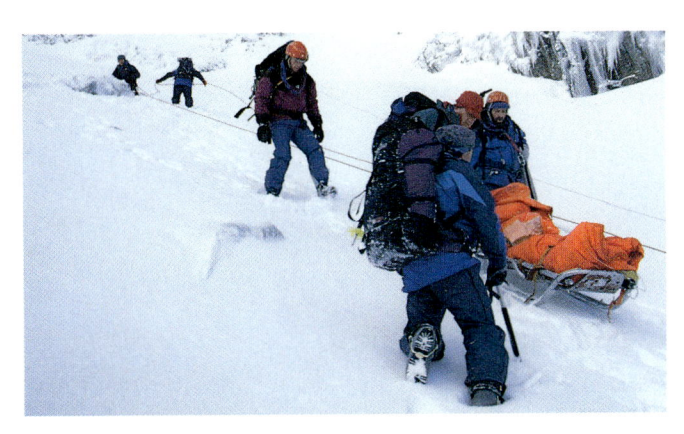

Other members of the team come to help lower the stretcher as the snow is extremely deep.

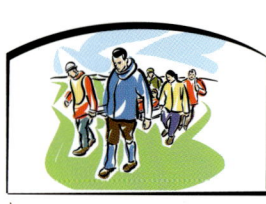

In an emergency

Avalanche warning

When there has been a heavy snowfall and teams are called out to a search, they have to be very aware of the risk of avalanches. Avalanches occur when the temperature has risen, when there is a sudden noise or vibration, and on steep slopes.

Teams are trained in avalanche rescues. Unlike other rescues, where a member of the climbing party might go to get help, it is vital to find the victim quickly. The rapid cooling of the victim plus the risks of suffocation and being crushed by the pressure of the snow reduce a person's chance of survival to 50 per cent after 30 minutes.

Using probes

The team is trained in the use of avalanche probes to locate people in

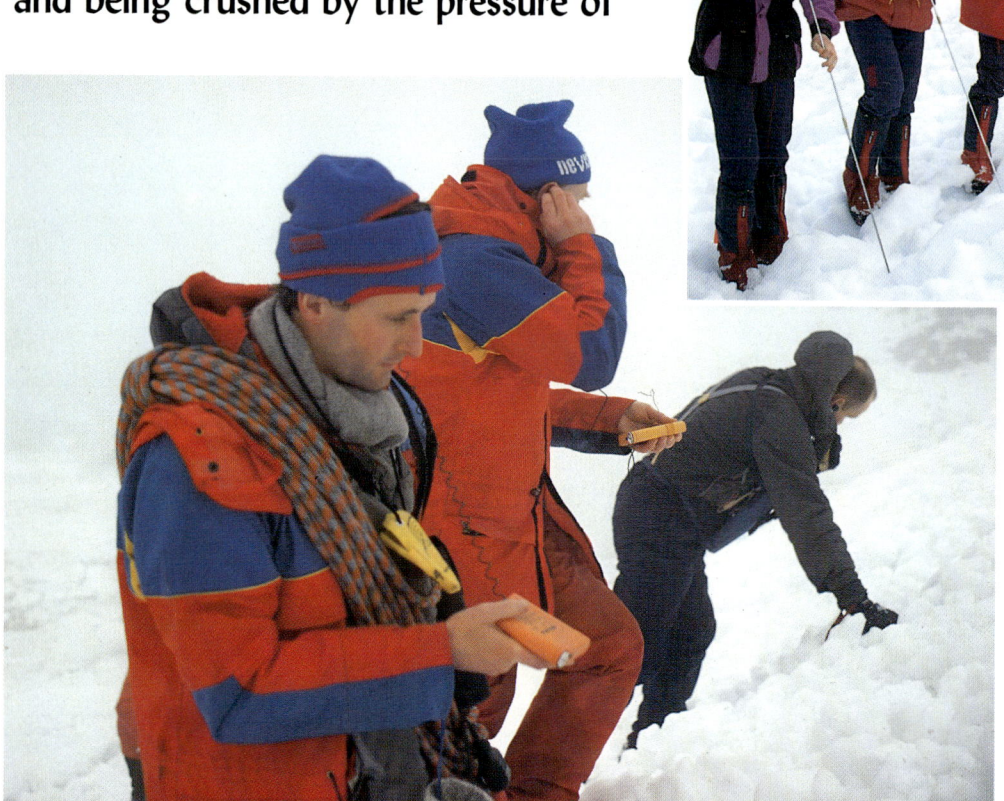

▲ Using avalanche probes.

◀ These members carry transceivers. If there is an avalanche the transceiver can pick up or give out a signal.

24

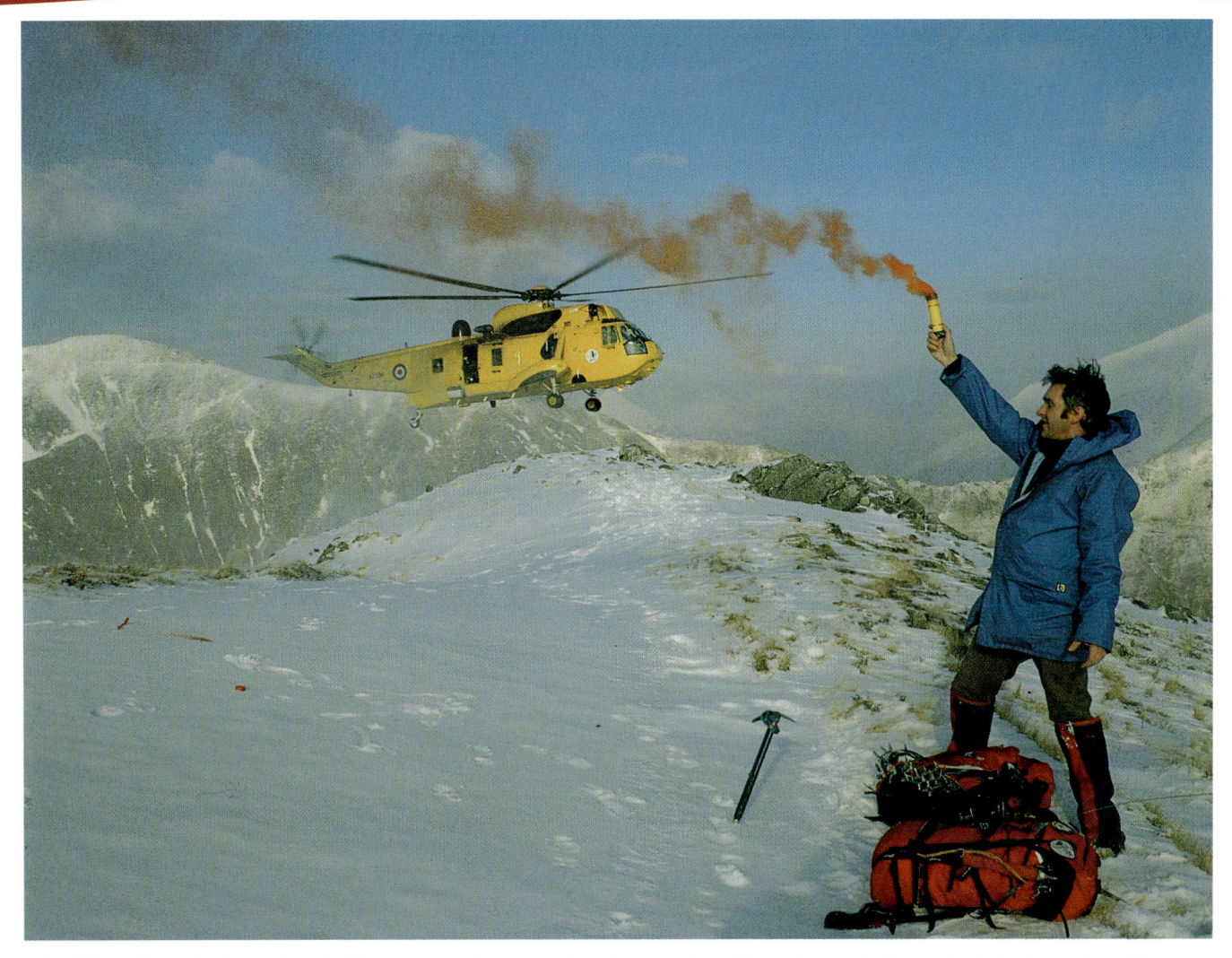

▲ The flare helps the helicopter pilot to check on the direction of the wind before landing or hovering. Usually the helicopter lands with the wind in front of it.

deep snow. Standing shoulder to shoulder each person pushes the probe into the snow three times before stepping forward – one push at each foot, and one between the feet.

Sending out flares

All teams carry flares. There are various types, but smoke flares are the most important. They are used to let the pilot of a helicopter know the direction and strength of the wind. It is difficult to spot someone on the mountain unless that person is moving. Letting off a flare gives a clear reference point to the crew. People setting off flares stand with their arms outstretched and the wind behind them so that the orange smoke does not blow into their faces. Each flare lasts for about three minutes.

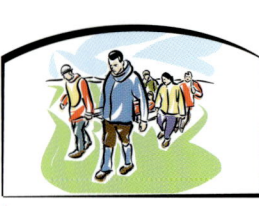

De-briefing

After every search or rescue I have a de-briefing with the team. Which parts of the rescue went well and why? Could we have done anything more efficiently? Did we have all the correct equipment to hand? When the casualty has recovered, we find out how he or she felt we had handled the situation. As a team we never stop learning and we are keen to improve our techniques.

▼ At the de-briefing discussion with the team, I make notes of any suggestions and comments for future rescues.

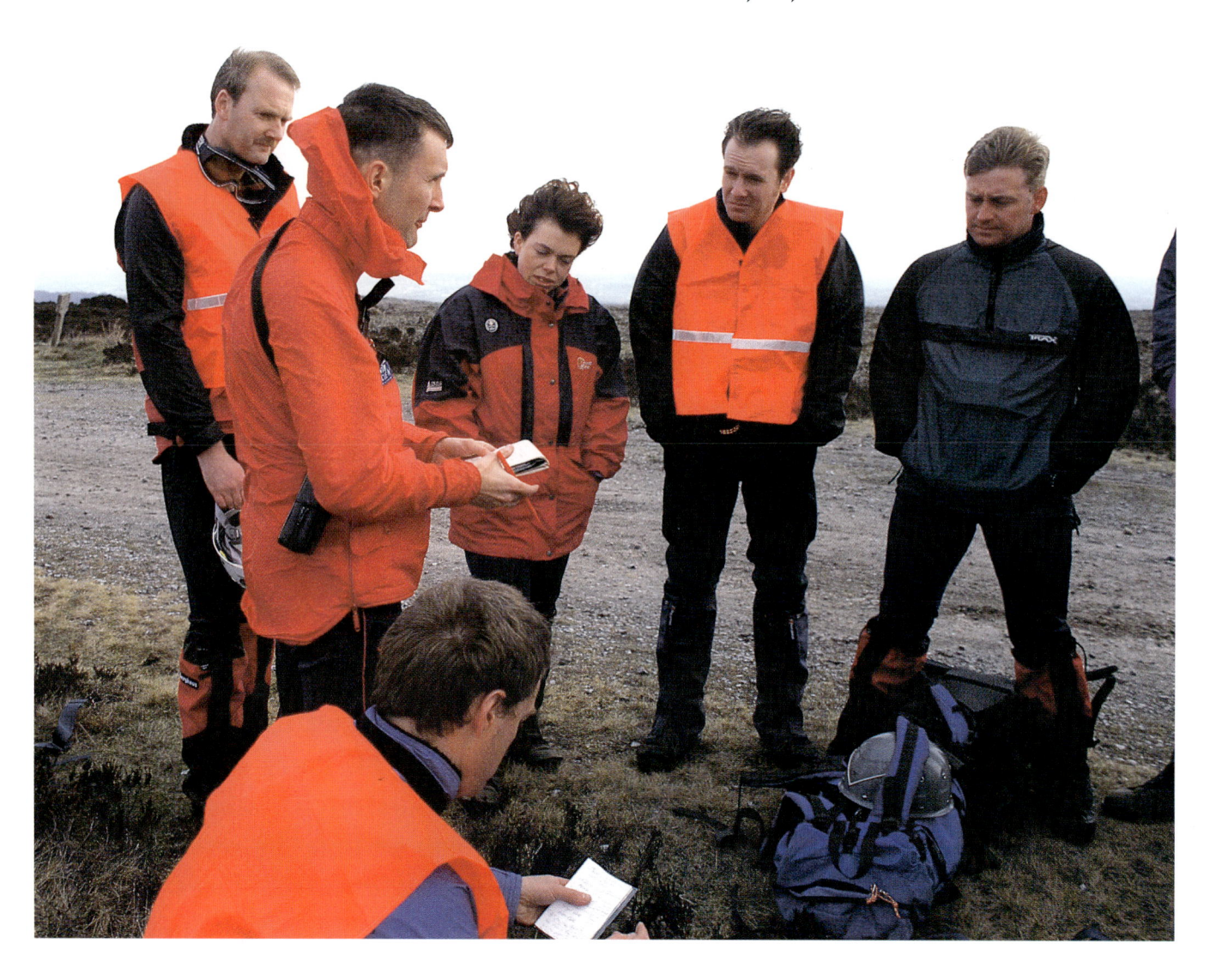

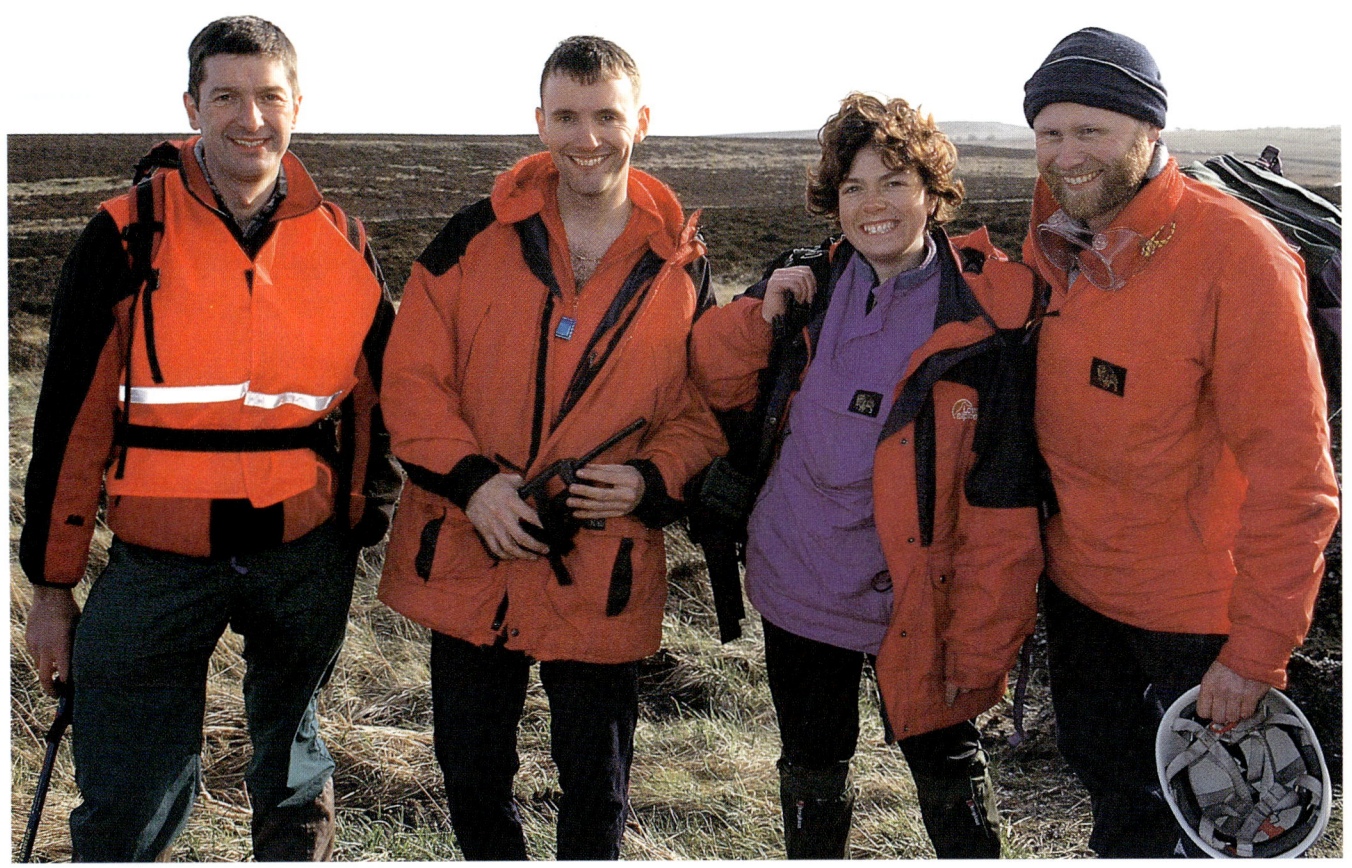

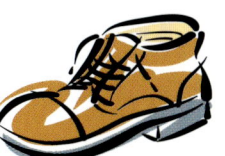

▲ We are all pleased because the rescue has gone well.

Safety points when out walking or climbing

- Make sure clothing is suitable for the conditions – windproof, warm and waterproof. Several layers of clothing are useful for insulation.
- Wear good walking boots.
- Tell people where you are going, your route and what time you expect to be back.
- Set off on your walk or climb at a sensible time, leaving plenty of time to return in daylight.
- Take a first-aid kit.
- Take a torch, spare bulbs and batteries.
- Take a whistle and know the signal for rescue – six long blasts and stop for a minute before repeating.
- Carry food and drinks – sweets, chocolates or glucose tablets provide extra energy.
- Carry a compass and walking map, and know how to use them.
- Carry a polythene survival bag for shelter.

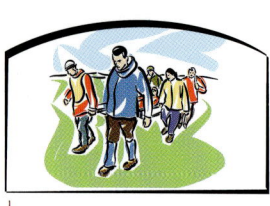

Glossary

bivouac bag a survival bag that provides protection from wind and rain in an emergency

box splint a padded splint for fixing a broken leg

crampons metal devices attached to the soles of climbing boots by straps to provide grip in icy conditions

gaiters coverings for the lower legs, from the instep of the foot to the knee; they are worn for protection from rain, wind, mud and snow

global positioning system a pocket-sized device that is used for accurate navigation; it uses a system based on satellite technology

gully a deep channel or small valley

handler the person who controls the dog on a search, usually the owner and trainer

hypothermia a condition that occurs when the body's temperature drops below 35°C; it is caused by exposure to cold, wet conditions or exhaustion

insulation a method of keeping warm by reducing heat loss

intravenous insertion of fluid into a vein

pager a small device used to contact another person by displaying a message on the screen, or by bleeping

paramedic a person who is trained to give emergency medical treatment

spindrift very fine frozen snow that drifts in the wind

splint a rigid device used to prevent the movement of a broken bone

strobe light a very bright light that flashes on and off

transceiver a radio device containing a transmitter and receiver which is used to detect victims of avalanches. The climbers at risk from an avalanche set the device to transmit a signal. If they are buried in an avalanche, searchers can set the device to receive the signal.

vacuum mattress a special mattress that moulds itself to the shape of a person; it is used to prevent movement on a stretcher

(to) winch to lift up with a rope or steel cable

Index

air scent 18, 20, 21
ambulance 10, 17, 21, 23
avalanches 24-25, 28

belay 14, 18
bivouac bag 22, 28
blood pressure 15
box splint 15, 28

call-out officer 8, 9
casualty bag 11, 15
clothing 11, 27
compass 11, 27
controller 8, 10, 11, 13, 17, 20
crampons 11, 22, 28

de-briefing 26
doctor 15
dogs 18-19, 20-21, 28

equipment 8, 11
exhaustion 23, 28

first aid 11, 12, 15, 27
flares 11, 25
food and drink 11, 27

gaiters 11, 28
global positioning system 11, 28
ground scent 21

handlers 18-19, 20-21, 28
helicopter 10, 14, 16, 17, 25
helmets 11
hospital 14, 17
hypothermia 15, 23, 28

ice axe 11, 22
insulation 15, 27, 28

maps 11, 12, 20, 27

oxygen 11, 23

pager 8, 11, 28
paramedics 16, 28
police 8, 10

radio check 10
radios 8, 12, 20, 28
ropes 11, 13, 14, 17, 28

shock 14, 23
spindrift 22, 28
splints 11, 15, 28
stretcher 11, 15, 16, 21, 23
survival bag 27, 28

transceiver 24, 28

vacuum mattress 11, 28

walking boots 11, 27
whistles 21, 27
winching 16-17, 28